The
Self Healing
Master in You

AnnaMarie Antoski

ISBN-13: 978-0-9868844-8-1

DEDICATION

CONTENTS

CONTENTS

ACKNOWLEDGMENTS

I acknowledge myself for my courage to continue the path of self healing and the trust it does take to sustain it long enough to experience the results.

I acknowledge You for taking the courageous steps that have energized this book to you. You are on your way to the powerful YOU through your experiences of self healing.

Chapter One

Defining Illness and Disease?

The most important part of all self healing is coming to the realization that it is your own self that has created the illness or disease to begin with. Yes I know that sounds like allot of responsibility, however you will find it to be so worth it when you experience you own self healing.

Illness and disease are words to describe a meaning for an experience of a body that is out of its natural harmony. Medical fields have created names to label

1

diseases to define any part of our body that has become out of ease. Not only have they come up with all these different names to label any disharmony in our body, they even create names for anything that pops up that can be boxed into creating it to be another disease. One that comes to mind is shyness. Whoever "they" who create the names to label any dysfunction is not important, the only importance is realizing these are just created names others have created to define a meaning to an experience that our body is out of its natural ease of harmony. In reference to shyness, when we realize that shyness is not a disease, it is a symptom that lacks self love for many reasons that it was originally created and sustained by the individual who experiences shyness. I believe that by labeling shyness as another disease, considering disease already has a bad wrap with many negative limiting and disempowering attachments that define it is creating more lack of wisdom about diseases in our body. So it's important to realize that definitions that label anything can also be dissected back to a neutral and loving state. A loving description that will remove fear thoughts regarding any disease creates it to be the best foundation to work with.

So throughout the book I will be referring to any illness as a disease. The reason being of the hidden meaning in the word itself that illuminates the seeded loving opportunity and resolution for the experience of disease. Disease when we hyphenate the word it reads dis-ease. Ease defines to be in flow, relaxed, in a peaceful state of being, when we add the "dis" in front of the word "ease" it becomes "disease" giving it a whole other meaning which simply means our body is out of ease of its natural flow of harmony.

I know this seems simple enough, however if you are experiencing any pain in your body, any illness or disease, then this simplicity has somehow been overlooked in your awareness. And is the very result of what you are experiencing presently because you have overlooked it to notice how out of your natural ease you have become. All you need to do is recall back in your memories of the times when you felt good, free of pain. You will realize that when you are free of pain, you feel good, you are at ease, which also means your body cells are at ease too. There is no disconnection of your body cells as being separate from you and your thoughts and feelings. Remembering that YOU are the one who is choosing the thoughts that created the disharmony originally and continues to create the disharmony in your body presently.

So it does become simple when you realize that any pain or disease in your body is your body cells way of communicating to you that you have allowed yourself to become out of your natural flowing ease of health.

This is all that disease is, not something to fear, instead it is a creation of experience subconsciously by you and for you to become aware how powerful you really are. You are so powerful that you can create disease from a body of cells of ease. That's powerful wouldn't you agree? It's that power that empowers you to realize when you really know that you created your disease that you can heal it too. It's only a reversal of choosing different thoughts that you have previously chosen and focus upon.

It's through the creation and experience of the disease that we become to learn how we actually created it. This brings us to become more consciously aware of how we are choosing to think on a daily basis. Questioning many old beliefs that dictate through illusions making it appear to define that everything just happens to us.

Creating disease is the greatest opportunity for us to know our selves more and take all of our power back. Power that we have been giving away to others, to our reactions, to illusions, to old beliefs and especially to our diseases.

So much of our power when we become diseased has been trickling bit by bit keeping us disempowered. This is the reason that defining the seemingly subtle messages that the body was trying to communicate but many do not listen until the disease becomes to the point of almost screaming in pain. To get you to finally notice what has been going on within yourself to begin with. Allowing you to finally understand what and how you have created the disease by what you have been entertaining too long with your thoughts and imaginings and verbal expressions of the story of yourself that you continue to keep telling and believing. That is really all it is, a story that you tell about yourself that keeps the spinning of your energy in the disease. How could you possibly heal when you continue to tell the same story of how you feel that you are getting worse and the pain is too? The secret to healing is to talk as if you are already on your way to healing. Act and feel as if you are healed so your body can pick up on the new commands. So let's continue to break it down in more detail of what disease really is.

Once we define what illness and disease really is, we then can take notice of what your body has been trying to tell you. When we keep in mind that our body's way of communicating is by giving us some signs that usually starts out subtly of a little discomfort. Yet for so many individuals these subtle signs go unnoticed. It's usually not until the dis-ease has become more noticeable that many then become aware of it.

An example is a small sniffle and runny nose starts and then weeks and then months go by and you notice it has developed into sinus infections. Then it seems to pop up whenever you are around certain things, or traffic or animals or even people, however people become easily disguised as other things. It all started this way and then you subconsciously associated certain things or people as an attachment. So you may even miss that you could be allowing others in your life to be affecting you and how you react to how they affect you is also creating irritations in your body ailments.

Connecting the Dots to See Through the Illusions

Connecting the dots is seeing through the illusions, in other words of what may appear to you as hidden beliefs. Another example that individuals body's are affected is by the season of spring and then there comes their belief that goes into re- action to create to bring on sinus attacks. Or it may be a belief in animal hair or types of fabric material and on and on the list is really endless of reasons all from beliefs that you became to value as a truth. You must become aware and ask yourself, how do you allow others or things or events or season to begin to affect you? It's from old programs, media conditioning and beliefs you carried on from well meaning other individuals.

Could it be another person triggering you to have an attack? Though it will always be the way we react to another or others that will be what triggers the so called "attack" it will appear in the illusion that it may be something that is attacking or happening to you. Keep in mind as a reminder that this is the illusion, the reality is that you are the one allowing the reaction of the creation of whatever it is you are believing is affecting you. Nothing and no one can really affect you unless you allow it which seems to occur without awareness that it is going on in the first place.

It does take deeper awareness to notice these subtle lingering signs and clues to be aware of. Any dis-ease or not feeling well may seem to pop up and becomes as if it's out of the blue, however there was always more time in the making or creating of it then it appears. It is usually something that has been bothering and irritating you for awhile that you did not realize until you feel pain or after the diagnosis. Many times it takes individuals being diagnosed with a disease and going through the healing stages before they connect the dots of how they created it to begin with, and the most important part is connecting the dots. It may take some practice in the beginning to notice the connection of your thoughts and illnesses before it becomes more habitual and easier.

This is the importance of being aware and noticing your reactions about everything because by changing your reactions, you can then change the creation of the disease or progressions of it.

A simple example I'd like to share with you is an awareness of experiences with mosquito bites. It has taken many occurrences for me to realize until I had experienced being a victim to the critters compared to not being a victim to them. I have been outside when others were getting bit all of over yet I had not experienced more then a couple buzzing around me and no bites on me. At the time I had been in blissful moods for weeks as I was so obsessed with experimenting on my thoughts to see the proof if they really are energy and create reality as I have read and read so much about. So for a few weeks this was a couple decades ago I was so aware as much as I could possibly be to transform all my negative reactions to positive responses. I was getting really good at it and started to notice how natural and habitual it was becoming after the first couple weeks of breaking the old automatic ways of past reacting. I could always know when I was making some new ground because of the way it became more instantly to respond differently then in the past.

Keep in mind also that throughout my whole life up to this point I have always been a magnet for bug bites. It did not matter when or where, if there were bugs, I would get bit or stung. You know the old saying that went something like, I must have the kind of blood that bugs like? Well I really believed it because I could see the evidence when I was outdoors. Now you can imagine my surprise when I watched others go through being massively bitten or stung when I was not. This is what made me ponder this for awhile to get to how the change could occur. And the only thing I could find was that my attitude had changed and of course when we change our attitude we change our inner body cells and blood and everything that goes along with it. Now a new belief had become reinforced for me that bugs do not like my blood as they did in the past.

This went on for a few years of no longer being stung or bitten by bugs until I went through some big challenges that I was not dealing with too well. All the years of work I had done on myself and when these challenges were in my path, even though I realized later that I created them for an exuberant reason, still it took me down for awhile. It allowed me to realize just how stubborn some of my hard nosed beliefs could be that they could resurface and I could become reacting to them as I did in my past. It was all for the reason that I stopped working on myself for awhile of being aware on a daily basis, which showed me that I needed to continue to do the work I was doing more consistently. It did not hard wire in my brain's memories to completely override the old beliefs, that was the reason I was reacting again in the old ways. One night a few friends and I were sitting outside by the fire pit and those critters were biting me and I could not take it. They were even going through my clothes.

This was a very big AHA moment and I sat that night and contemplated it all.

To have the experience of being bitten for years then not being bit for years was no coincidence. Considering even at the time I knew everything is energy and when we change our thoughts we change our attitude and that changes everything, even if it's back to the old ways again.

My blood and body had changed again by my reactions to the new challenges that I was handling the old ways. By complaining and wondering why me? After my few hours alone in my own reflection of it all I told myself this is it, it's the new way from now on. This is only one example, I could write hundreds of pages of experiences of all kinds that I have went through, some major ones and others smaller ones. For me it was the combination of the awareness on a consistent basis that continued to show me over and over again all the proof from all the experiences. I will share a few of these experiences throughout this book.

Back to the bug bites, so my thoughts changed and my attitude changed, which then changed the reality I experience. Whenever I was a magnet to bites or stings were the times when I felt like a victim in my own reality by reacting disempowering, as if I have no control over my experiences. I was reacting negatively to the challenges I was going through and creating my own victim mentality by the thoughts I was choosing without awareness that I kept thinking. When I no longer experienced being a magnet to bites and stings, I did not feel like a victim, I actually felt empowered because I was constantly transforming my thoughts that created good feelings and was responding differently about everything. Especially the things and individuals that bothered me the most. I realized absolutely that thoughts really are energy, they are things. How I think and then feel creates how I react or respond to everything and it makes a huge difference in my body too.

That is the reason I said that this is only a simple experience of bug bites however it was so profound that it inspired me to continue this amazing journey of self awareness and the nature of reality and self healing. I love the quote in the movie, "What the Bleep Do We Know" about thoughts and water, "If words can do that to water, imagine what it can do to our body?" That was another revelation, more proof that thoughts do matter and create matter in reality in every way and is the reason I have been self healing for over twenty years.

Another experience that also inspired me to continue the self healing journey was again decades ago when I became divorced. At the time I could not understand how I became sickly for years with all kinds of heart problems and sinus and lung infections until after I separated from my marriage, it was as if I was instantaneously healed. What is referred to as miraculous healing and this also urged me to question so many things which also lead me on my self healing path. I wanted to know how all these symptoms I had suffered with for years all of a sudden just seem to disappear. I also appeared younger physically too. To shorten the whole story what I had found from all my research about the nature of reality and our body's connection gave me all the answers I was wondering so much about.

Simply I became not happy in my marriage and when my husband wanted a reason for the separation, all that came out of me was I wanted to find myself. Even back then I had no idea what I was searching for, it sounded crazy even to him. Looking back at it all now I can see exactly the reasons and I was on a path of discovery not only more about myself but about life and the nature of reality, beliefs and how it affects everything including my body and much more. It didn't have anything to do with my husband, it had everything to do with me and the freedom and experiences I needed to go through to learn and continue evolving. I had also read many books and heard from others who also had said the same thing, they needed to find themselves. All finding ourselves really means is getting to know more about who we really are and how and why we choose to think the thoughts we think that affects everything.

Which leads us to the realization of how powerful we really are and that we are a creator creating reality and our body by the thoughts we choose that create the emotions we feel.

So I was sickly for years because I became unhappy because I just thought there had to be more to life then just a routine marriage and raising children. I became stuck for too long and that created quite the victim mentality for too long that my body was then reacting and becoming sicker. When I separated from my marriage and became independent, I became happy and felt free with no conditions or control and everyday I was learning and experiencing so much more even through all the hard challenges I was going through. My learning became my passion and I was constantly reading, learning for years and still do. I found the answers and the connections, when I stayed consistently joyful my body responded from it all with no longer being sick. You will read in the last chapter that research has now shown that being in joy and bliss and literally has a affect on our body cells, heart and affects the changes in our DNA.

I am not suggesting either way which way is the best to becoming joyful, it can be done by staying in a marriage and working on your own self. Using all of it as an opportunity instead of an escape goat, that is your own personal choice and decision. Knowing what I know now, maybe I would have done that and am actually doing that in my present relationship. The important part in all of this is knowing that being joyful no matter what is going on is what sustains your body to respond by creating a healthy body. Self love and being joyful no matter what is going on is ease and harmony in the body just because it's a natural state. Meaning that it can not be conditional or dependant on anything else, if it is then it's being happy. And being happy creates highs and lows because it keeps us dependant on something outside of us. that is going on, it will always come back to yourself and how you respond.

A Very Important Powerful Question

Just as I asked myself in my past, I now ask you this very important question, do you want to stay a victim and sick? Or would you rather be empowered and healed?

You are going to be one way or the other, the only difference is the empowering way will take some effort until it becomes natural and trusted through your own experiences. At first it may seem very challenging but the most important part is not giving up no matter what you have to go through. This is a very crucial stage you will go through because you will be creating new beliefs to override the old ones. Reminding yourself often that you are greater then you pain, you are greater then you disease, you are stronger and will not only heal yourself you will know yourself and that leads you on the most fascinating empowering evolving journey of all. Believe me it is so worth it!

Onward we go healing lovers, the battle may seem as if it has just begun, however it is now coming to an end. No more fighting against disease, instead you are going to embrace and love the disease for all it can show you as you expand and grow exuberantly as a result of your disease. Then you are going to heal it by your knowledge into your wisdom from your amazing experiences.

Chapter Two

My Own
Experiences
Of Self Healing

The reason I am writing and explaining about the power of self healing is because I have been healing myself for over twenty years. I am writing from my own experiences to share with you who is reading this book presently. You have this book in your hand right now because you are taking your power back and you are courageous enough once and for all get to the root of your disease or illness. I want to share how empowering self healing really is when you give it the attention and experience it repetitiously, then you will also know how empowering self healing is for you. Unfortunately they do not give out doctoral degrees or any type of recognition that I can label myself as an authority because self healing is still out of the norm. Though there are more then there ever was in the past that are self healing, it is still not in the mainstream of being a safe and most effective way to heal any or all diseases. Yet it is the safest and most natural way to heal. This is a powerful reason that you should really congratulate yourself for taking this leading edge journey into self healing. You will find through each self healing success that you experience the power that has been available all along to you will melt all doubt away.

I do consider myself a great authority because I have been doing it for so long. Just as any and all self healers will also confirm to the fact that self healing is the most empowering experiences for our selves and also in guiding others too. There is no negative side affects because it's so natural and how our body was designed to work originally.

Though I still consider myself to continually be on a journey of evolving stages of learning and experiencing creating my reality and every single part of it, I consider myself to be a great authority on self healing. I am evolving in a sense that just as we grow up in physical as babies and we learn and grow through different stages into finally adulthood. Then it seems once we become adults we then have the graceful opportunity which I believe is an urging of our infinite spirit to evolve even further. To awakening into spiritual wisdom and grow while evolving to combine spiritual into physical with awareness. Which I love to refer to as Infinite Beingness.

So it has been over twenty years of my own learning experiences through experimenting and then relearning through perpetual growth. While evolving through stages into what could now be perceived as my teenage spiritual stages evolving into an adult aware graceful creator in my being unifying spiritual into physical.

So do I still create illnesses or dis-eases for myself? Yes, not as often as in my past and it becomes almost rare however I still miscreate to learn more as a result. Sometimes the illnesses even becomes greater because I believe I have even greater experiences to learn as I bring my body back to health or ease quicker. For the reason that I already have quite the stack of memories to retrieve of my successes of self healing is the reason that it becomes that if I do miscreate I can quickly realign my body back to harmony quicker then ever. This is how it creates the healing to be so quick. Once I go through whatever it was I subconsciously created then I also excel to evolve even greater in my spiritual evolution in embodiment. To me no disease is big or even incurable anymore, all disease is only a disharmony of the body from its natural ease. Now doesn't that take allot of pressure of stress right off the get go? And when I sustain my love and joyfulness completely, all the time, there will no longer be anymore miscreating either.

When I first began and was experimenting with the idea of self healing which I was learning from many great teachers and their teaching of information. I was experiencing repetitiously migraines, lung infections, sinus, irritations, allergies, back pain and even heart problems. Along with long bouts of depression that would last for weeks before I would finally experience a week absence of depression before depression would take me over for another 3 weeks. I was only in my twenties of age, so young and so sickly, this was the time I spoke of in the first chapter about my unhappy years in my marriage but it started even earlier.

I had carried these beliefs and attitudes from my teenage years. I had created gull bladder problems with gull stones and experienced weeks of excruciating painful attacks before they finally removed my whole gull bladder. The doctor told me that I would never be able to eat greasy food again. Well even though at that time I did not know about self healing or creations of disease, I did believe the doctors were wrong. I was always a rebel and felt so uncomfortable with rules, which I can now see is actually an evolving way to be. I believed that I would be able to eat whatever I wanted and not be affected by not having a gull bladder. I even secretly believed my gull bladder would grow back. Ever since those days and still to this day I can eat anything I want and am not affected by any pain or dysfunction of it at all.

Since I do not use the medical field of doctors or hospitals I have never been checked to see if a new gull bladder has been produced into creation in my body, I just believe it is. Though I no longer had any problems with my gull bladder I did continue my sickly patterns of illnesses for a couple more decades before I came upon self healing.

Back then I believed that everything happen to me and had no idea that I created my reality, except for setting goals that many times I did not accomplish very quick either. Of course when I look back through hindsight now, it is so obvious how and even the reason why I was creating all the pain and dis-ease I was experiencing. But I learned massively in the next thirty years that would follow. If I looked back as a future being to consolidate that younger version of myself I could have excelled so much quicker. As it's stated, there's a reason for everything we go through, so it was the journey I needed for my evolution of my soul. This is also something to consider which I do presently by having an open connection to my future or infinite self. Yet for many in their younger years the interest of self healing or wisdom of creating our reality is not enhanced enough that they want to know. Except for "psychic kids" self healing seems to still be in the minority of humanity's collective consciousness.

Other healings I have experienced is growing my hair back when I had unconsciously created bald spots in two different times in my life. A result of anxiety and stress which I didn't know about back then. Now it's recognized that stress creates all havoc and disharmony in our body. I have also experienced eye vision improved too. If I created a migraine I was able to just put my hand on my head and the pain is gone within minutes. I rarely create headaches or migraines now.

So for you who have found your way to this book, I congratulate you big time on your courage to break free of the mainstream illusions. I guarantee you when you are ready for self healing, you will be amazed how empowering and inspiring it is in every area of your life. It will open the door to even more then you could ever have imagined.

Reminding yourself often of the wisdom that You Can Trust Yourself, that you were actually designed, your body was created to trust your own self. You really are the best authority regardless of what the mainstream media or medical field may dictate. Your loving intuition will guide you to the most powerful wisdom, all you have to do is practice listening to that wisdom of knowledge and then trust it. Through practice I guarantee you that you will come to the same awareness and agreement.

One more important thing I would like to mention is that I do not use any herbal or natural health food or anything for that matter for healing. The only thing I use is my own thinking and feeling to do the work. If I want to use something, I pick something, example chocolate almonds and create them to be a healing helper. I enjoy creating my own things and give them the power by my thoughts when I desire to be creative. For me I know that it is not what we consume, it is always what we THINK about what we are putting in our mouth or body that creates the way our body will react. This is what sustained me from using anything but the power of my thoughts and feelings to direct my body to do what it does best, take my commands. This is the reason that I repetitiously mention the power is in you, you are the one that chooses either consciously or without awareness of how everything will affect you.

The self healing master is inside you, always has been and will always be, the only difference is being aware of yourself as the master. Remind yourself often that everything really is neutral when you remove all attached judgments from your beliefs about everything. By doing this you can choose to give power to anything with awareness that you are doing it and that is a powerful state to be in.

You will notice repetition in many of the powerful ideas throughout this book and it is for a very good reason. While reading through the whole book you will be reprogramming your new beliefs while you read, similar to affirmations. So it is a very powerful and great creating reason for the repetition as it adds to create new memories even as you read you are creating new memories and empowering yourself.

Now let's go forward into knowing more about our body.

Chapter Three

Your Body, Your Living Organism

Let us take a deeper look at our body. Our body appear to be a solid unit of being contained within it of organs, cells, spine, nervous system and a brain. That is the most simplistic definition of our body. We use it to live our day to day life, in other words it gets us around. When we take it for granted that our body is just a body without going deeper to realize that it is so much more magnificent then ever realized before any disease. When we realize our magnificence of our bodies then we can observe disease in the most loving of light. In rays of not only hopeful optimism, but also in rays of love and empowerment for the opportunity that the disease had shown us that we learn from it as a result.

When we go deeper while we expand our mind or consciousness we come to realize what our body really is. Data of research has shown that our body is a living organism of over 70 trillions individual cells that are responding to what we think about most of the time. Again it's so worth repeating, actually read the next paragraph out loud a couple times as you let your mind ponder and really absorb the wisdom of how exuberant this information really is.

My body is my living organism of over 70 trillion individual cells working together to create the physical body that I experience.

Now how magnificent is this that our body is a living organism of over 70 trillion body cells that are individual yet they work together? So they either work together to create a great healthy feeling body or working together to create an ill diseased body. All dependent on what you choose to think that triggers you to then feel that programs your brain while simultaneously all other parts of your body's nervous system, molecules, proteins are also working together too. All of this orchestrated together that creates your body that you experience every day in every way. Now doesn't that change the way you perceive the power of You and your body?

This deeper comprehension allows us to realize to know that our body is not just a machine working along and that everything just somehow happens to it.

This illusion that defines to dictate that diseases just happens to us and if we take a pill it will take care of everything. These types of beliefs limit us in so many ways so that we miss the greatest opportunities to know who we really are and how our body actually functions.

Let's use the analogy of a band aid when we cut our finger. We cut our finger and we clean the cut with whatever disinfectant we use and then we place a band aid on the cut and go about our day. We know it's an illusion to think that the band aid itself is healing the cut, right? We know it's not the band aid that is doing the healing, the band aid is only protecting the cut from any dirt getting into it. So in a sense we could see the band aid as having a connection of an affect to our healing of our cut. Yet deeper we know that even if we did not have a band aid available, our cut would still heal. We would have to be more careful not to allow dirt to get on the cut. It is our body's natural healing ability that continues to heal the cut in our skin and all the cells in that area come together from the signal to heal, ease the cut back to harmony of the healing naturally.

So this analogy can show us that just as we do not believe the band aid is the healer, yet we have been conditioned hypnotically to believe that a pill, like the band aid is healing us. Seeing it in this light we can realize how easily we can be deceived into believing that anything other then our own self can be the real healer. When that is the farthest from the genuine reality of what is really going on. Our body's natural way is to heal when we get out of the way when we think thoughts that are no longer denying the body's ability to heal. The ability to heal is always there, it is the thoughts we keep choosing to think that redirects the body to continue the disease. Yes, go ahead and read that last sentence again, it's very powerful to absorb.

As we continue to focus and imagine in our mind when we first cut our finger and the cut in the skin is now open and cells gather together to do what they naturally are programmed to do, heal. Blood gushes outward and what is that blood doing? It is the body's natural disinfecting ingredients that is cleaning the wound of any infectious particles. Then all the cells that gathered about to do their natural work continue by allowing the atmosphere of natural air to sew up the spot that then closes it up. It really takes care of itself when we allow it to do what it does best, self heal. When we get in the way of the cut's healing we we think thoughts of fear that the cut may get infected. When we

27

continue to think in fears energy, we then will create the commands to the body cells that will create infection. That is how we can get in the way of all healings, to get out of the way is to think loving trustful thoughts and just let go and allow the cells to heal the cut. Whether we choose to be aware of this powerful wisdom or not we will be creating either getting in the way by commanding by our thoughts to create infection or getting out of the way and creating healing.

There is no difference in the example of a cut in comparison to any disease, especially diseases that have been labeled as curable or not. All diseases are curable except if the individual has the belief that is dictating it not to be, and even that is flexible enough to change too.

When we think about and imagine that we are the instructor, we are the one in control to conduct a symphony of 70 trillion cells all depending on our beliefs and how we choose to think that creates how we feel. When we come to know that our beliefs are only bunched up thoughts that we have thought about and valued long enough that have become what we believe about everything and anything. That is how flexible and changeable our beliefs really are and we can always create new beliefs by thinking newer thoughts. Any new thoughts thought over and over again will become the new belief that will then support the new you, the new reality and the new way the body will take its instructions.

So again let's regurgitate fear versus love thoughts about a cut, we have the choice to infect the cut with our doubtful fearful thoughts. If we do that then we will experience our cut to become eventually infected. Who infected the cut? The one who continued the fearful doubting thoughts gave the message for those cells that were already in the process to heal the cut originally has now taken new directions to infect it now. You gave it the instructions by what you focused your thoughts about, what you talked about, how you see it to be. Nothing outside of you gave your body cells the instructions, it has been you all along.

Even if your old programs of beliefs try to deny this or try to influence your thoughts to doubting this, then use that doubt as the biggest opportunity to correct that kind of thinking. Instead perpetually tell yourself that you are the power, you are the one, the master that has always been and is in control of the thoughts you want to think and talk about. Watch for little proofs of evidence in your life, even at first if it is small experiences, it is still proof and eventually evidential memories of proof will build up so that you have more memories to retrieve as a result.

Observe by your self awareness even if it's by looking through hindsight how things that irritated you that you kept inside has now created an infection. Then notice where in the body the infection is located because that will show you where you have stored emotions that have become blocked. If it is an infection in your hand? Focus for the answers to come to you, could it be there is something you may not like to be doing that you use your hands daily? Is the infection in your mouth? Then what is it you may be denying that you are not verbally expressing or mentally expressing? Is it in your bladder? What may be really pissing you off, creating the anger that you are not dealing with? This is just a few examples and you can use these types of examples with every disease, discomfort, pain or illness that you are feeling. Dig deeper to allow the connections to be shown to you, to come through to you, and it will when you ponder it deeper with more focus and trust that the wisdom will be revealed to you.

The body and all its cells never judges, it only responds to what we tell it by what we choose to think.

So now I am quite sure that you do realize and appreciate the grand master role you are to your magnificent living organism which is your body and how you are the one commanding the creation. If the realization of this knowing has not set it yet, then at least you are on your way.

Let us take an even deeper look at how we can recreate anything to be healed. Our body actually lives in the past and is a result of what we have been thinking and feeling prior to this present moment.

So our desire is to heal whatever we have created to be out of harmony in our body. The life we are living are experiences. The knowledge that any experience we have creates a memory and all emotions are a result of an experience.

Knowing this is a great advantage, however we need to take this knowledge now into our own experiences for it to become our own wisdom. Then this wisdom is literally creating the new memories from your new experience of healing even one ailment in your body. It's enough to create new memories to retrieve over the older ones that kept you in a limited loop. This can only be done by working it yourself through consistent awareness and practicing until a new experience that you have healed something that was an illness, pain or disease. When you do it once you create a new memory from the experience with a new emotion attached to that new memory.

When you heal another ailment, you have another experience that creates another memory containing trust and mastery, making it easier for the next healing to occur. By consistently doing this you are breaking the old loop you were stuck which is also where emotional energy has been stored in a certain spot in your body. Now you are creating new empowering memories to retrieve of your successes. This also unblocks the emotional energy that was blocked and releases the energy to flow. Think of it as a dam that has blocked your healing or any area of your life you feel stuck in.

Eventually you will find that anytime you feel pain, discomfort or illness or disease, it become easier to believe that you are the master of your body. You gain more and more trust and healing power. You literally become a new person with new memories and emotional feelings with the greatest potential of new beliefs. It then become second nature and the master healer has awakened and is alert and in control now.

In the beginning stages, more knowledge still needs to be learned to convince the old personality that keeps trying to urge you back in the comfort zone of disempowerment.

So onward we go to decipher what your body has been trying to tell you before your disease became to worsen. All for the reason you were not listening to begin with, once you do start to listen by being aware of how you are feeling, the deciphering begins.

Chapter Four

What is
Your Body
Telling You?

Your body is a magnificent wonderful communicator that will always inform you of what is going on with you. If you are feeling no pain that is the body's communication that all is great. That means the thoughts you have been choosing whether aware or not, but hopefully by now you are keeping yourself more aware then not aware. So you are noticing most of the time what your body is communicating on an on going basis. So the good feeling is your body telling you in the only way it can by how you feel that the thoughts you have been choosing to think have been hopeful, loving, light, free, positive, optimistic and more carefree. You know those high vibration thoughts that contain within them to trigger those good feelings.

There is really not much difference when you are feeling pain except for the difference of the emotions you are feeling. The body is still communicating to you but now it is communicating hurt, pain to give you the message that something has become out of harmony of your body's natural flow. Hmm could it be that for awhile you started thinking about something that is stressing you out? Detouring you from your joyful state into a fearful loop of memories and leads you to feeling nervous or anxious or a frustrated worried state?

For example you were thinking about how great it is that you have been feeling really good for hours, no pain. Then within a twinkling of a second or minute, you probably lost track of time and didn't even notice until you resurrect the reminiscing of how you even detoured. However you catch it by realizing you were feeling great until you started to wonder about the reasons that you feel so good when a few hours ago you were in pain. That is all it takes, a few minutes of pondering and wondering in your imagination as thoughts start to pop up about doubting and then fear will creep in so subtly and next thing you realize you are feeling fatigued. Then you start to feel the pain resurfacing again, which becomes attached to more choosing of thoughts and the downward spiral of pain resurfaces more intensely now.

All we have to do is consider realizing that it was us all along that have been orchestrating this symphony of body cells to take another route, the path of creating dependent on our thoughts focused again.

This is so empowering because it keeps showing us the more we become aware and become even excited about the knowledge that we are creating it all sustains more good feelings. What a game of adult hide and seek we play with illusion of beliefs.

I found it so exciting and amazing when I came to this realization that it has been me all along! This is so empowering because there is no one left to blame, only myself and then to release all blame into awareness.

Awareness is always a good thing when we perceive all learning experiences this way.

When I came to also realize that blaming myself is only a stage that we can sit in longer or just pass right through it. Blaming will only alter healing. It is when we take full responsibility for what our body is communicating to us and then choose new thoughts that will be beneficial to our healing instead of detouring and creating more pain and disease. This is the most powerful reason for excitement, joy, fun, laughter, bliss and love while simultaneously progressing on the self healing journey through all experiences you go through.

So we become excited because we realize we are so powerful that we create disease to bring us to awareness that it's our own self creating it all. Then we revel in self laughter of how comical it really is, simple but true, and how creative we really are in our creations. Then it brings us to joy and optimism because we can take all that power and realign it with new potential thoughts to focus and imagine starting to feel the healing begin. As long as we continue to choose better thoughts and insert better thoughts every time we notice the old fear thought surfacing, we will be on our way to being healed.

You will no longer be stuck in the fog lost and confused of what your body is telling you. If you have a pain, you ask yourself, what have you been thinking about or have you been judging yourself or your circumstances in something for too long? What's been bothering you for awhile that you have kept inside or talked verbally about long enough that the body cells reacted to the message and has now created as body pain? Remember your body cells are just doing their job, reacting by responding to what you are thinking and feelings and saying. They never judge anything, they only perform by your command.

How do you then heal an infection? By choosing to decipher the meaning of what's infecting (affecting) you. Whatever is bothering you, make peace with it.

Is it really worth playing more in the alteration of being bothered by anything or anyone when you know your body is going to react with creating pain?

I am quite sure you are answering no, nothing is worth being in this much pain about. So to be at peace with anyone or anything that bothers you is to let it go by forgiving it. Yes, that's the final stage of allowing the healing process to takes its cue of command.

Transform it All to Peace

Forgiving whether it is our self or another person for whatever they have done that bothered us, forgiving a situation, whatever it is, forgive it so that peace can be brought back into play instead of playing around with negative thoughts. The longer we linger in the negative energy the longer it will be before we start to feel better. Many times this powerful stage may go unnoticed, when you feel better just because someone else you were in conversation with talked about some happy things. So there can be many things that will be temporary for peace to resurface, however it's getting to the root of it all that actually creates the healing to be complete so that it doesn't resurface consistently. We have all heard of people that become cured or healed of cancer then years later it may appear again. The reason it reappears is because the root belief that creates the attitude they feel has not been completely changed for the new healthy sustained brain and body to sustain the new health.

That is what forgiving actually does in a deeper root part of us as it flows through our hearts into all of our body cells so that our cells can respond of their natural harmony.

Whenever you are feeling anything other then feeling great is when you can realize and become more aware of what you body is telling you. It has no other way of communicating to you to get your attention then by allowing the feeling of disharmony to surface. If any pain intensifies then all that is going on is that you have not paid attention enough yet. So the pain will increase and increase more, so will the disease until IT, the body's communication is finally reciprocated and you get the message so clearly.

Sore throat, suppressed emotions from thoughts pondered too long, cells gather together clumping up causing an energy blockage. Throat area represents your vocal expression. The soreness gets your attention, your throat hurts, again what's been bothering you? Work on letting it go, write a letter but don't mail it, speak to another who you trust that will just listen and also let it go. Whatever way you choose to allow it to become unblocked by letting whatever is bothering you out, will all come down to letting those bothersome thoughts eventually go. Then continue by seeing your throat already healed and feeling better and better and then back to the natural feeling of harmony.

I am not going to pretend that this is an easy thing to do in the beginning of self healing because of old beliefs and programs of memories of old reactions that have become so habitual. At first it may even seen impossible. It may take days or weeks in the beginning to override the old beliefs long enough to create a strong belief system to support the new ideas of self healing and the trust that finally comes from the enduring. When you heal yourself once, then twice and so forth, you now have newer memories to retrieve that will make it easier in future self healings. Your brain is actually rewiring the new memories for your retrieval and pushing further back the older memories.

You can do this with everything, every area of your body that you feel pain or discomfort or disease. Whatever area the pain is coming from is already a result of harboring thoughts that went unnoticed for too long. Bring yourself back to the powerful present moment with awareness and choose potentially better thoughts and reactions.

You must remind yourself consistently that your body is never judging, it is only responding to your thoughts, that your body cells take all commands from YOU. Then your body creates the disharmony, pain or disease, or harmony, ease of no pain.

Finally accepting to believe into knowing that your body is always communicating depending on what you are thinking long enough that becomes your beliefs. 70 trillion cells working continuously by reproducing and responding to whatever you are thinking, feeling and talking about long enough.

Chapter Five

Disease
as a Sign Post
to Change Directions

Disease as you now have come to realize to know is only a communication from your body to get your attention that if you do not makes some changes, the disease will worsen. It really has no other choice because if you do not heed the calling of the body's communication then it continues to perform from your commands.

Those commands of thoughts are a result of old ways of thinking, speaking and behaving and if you do not get the message then the pain will become louder which is similar to the pain screaming at you. Louder in the way of it worsening through more intensified pain. Even what is labeled as silent killers, seemingly no symptoms evident, there are always symptoms to be noticed even if they are so subtle. It takes precise awareness to sometimes fine tune the body's communication but it will always show you sign posts along the way.

Whatever the disease of pain experienced in the body can be perceived analogist as sign posts. Anywhere we travel there are directional signs, whether its street signs, city or town signs, they are there for a good reason. As we travel we are guided to continue in the direction that will take us to our destination. Disease can be perceived the same way. It may appear as a disease that somehow came out of the blue but that is an illusion, a disease starts and progresses if we have not notice the signaling as a sign post that will always try to get our attention.

So you are living your life, kind of happily it seems then all of a sudden you get the results of a disease. It's that "kind of" that may go so unnoticed. The great knowledge is that the disease is the end result, however it can also be a new beginning too. The disease can be the sign post along your journey of life to get your attention to change the direction you were going.

An example is cancer, it is the end result of a body system that was functioning harmoniously until some inserted daily thoughts pondered upon too long was the added ingredients that activate the havoc. Whether it was someone or situation that happened years ago, whenever the thought of it comes up there is still some resentment. Some unfinished business with either judgments on yourself or others or situations, places or things. You may notice throughout the years you just let these kinds of resentments, anger, frustrations and so on go as you went on with other things. However, so subtly throughout the years every time thoughts about the person or the situation or whatever it is has popped up you have never really dealt with it. You have just passed it off but the volcano has been brewing so deeply but has not erupted yet. The eruption finally burst when the disease is found, it has been brewing a long time and every time you added more fuel to it. And without noticing it either because you did not know previously about all of this knowledge, that's the reason you are reading this book or you just didn't desire to deal with it.

Be easy on yourself and be grateful with appreciation while loving yourself to finally have come upon the courage to know now or to do something about it now. You will find that nothing is worth altering your self love for but until you do realize it, these signs of disease will be the greatest opportunities to change your direction. I am not saying that it will not take some work, however if you are really ready to change directions with your thoughts, it will become a great adventure of experiences. Passion may even insert itself into the mix and when it does, passion will sustain anything and everything you will have to do to get your to healing.

The disease of cancer is one sign post, so is a heart attack or back injury's or any disease, too many to even mention, but if it's a disease, it's only an opposite direction that always has the power in itself to be changed. Just as all sign posts are used for as a directional indicator to change roads if you want to get to your destination. And what is everyone's natural destination to get to being once they have had enough experiences of what they do not want, so they can then experience what they do want, free of pain and disease? To enjoy life with a peaceful ease, in other words to be joyfully blissfully happy. So we can read DISEASE as a SIGN POST, the sign post reads, **YOUR POWER IS NOW, CHANGE DIRECTION.**

When we follow that sign, we then choose to change our old direction we have been creating from old thoughts to a new direction of new thoughts. We learn to know that the power is now, in this moment or any moment we choose or when we are ready to choose will be the POWERFUL MOMENT. The moment when we let go and surrender to the old ways of thinking that created not feeling good body communication. We embrace the powerful moment into a repetitious momentum to continue with the new empowering ways to think. Then we are on a different road, a different journey in new ways and our body cells take their new commends and start creating a body ease, instead of disease.

Chapter Six

Importance of Beliefs
In
HEALING

Knowledge about beliefs is important because if you are not aware of what you believe your body will continue to create the discomfort, pain or disease. When you do heal yourself irrelevant of time that may pass, if your beliefs have not changed, either will your old attitude and the disease will return. Beliefs are what creates our reality, whether you believe it or not, this is how reality is created. Beliefs are bunched together thoughts however those bunched up thoughts that create our belief systems can be very stubborn as a result of valuing them for so long. Whether you have carried your beliefs from past conditioning or any conditioning that limits your power, beliefs can be picked up from all different sources.

Television supplies many suggestions that become beliefs as you watch programs and advertisements. Data of information is perpetually picked up and most of the time we are not aware of the process that is going on as those suggestions are creating memories in our brain. Many beliefs were conditioned from birth and continued throughout your life. It is not important where the conditioning of your beliefs have come from, the most important point is that you are aware of what your beliefs are because they have created many different attitudes about everything.

Usually when finding out you have a disease many beliefs are already in the process of changing as you start to question yourself and disease in general. All the questioning of why me? What did I do wrong? Many wonderings start to get the ball rolling aligning you in a different direction than before the disease. However it may not get to all the beliefs but it starts to form a different pattern of thinking.

A belief is thoughts that has been gathered together and created a system that you have subconsciously without awareness, or consciously with awareness have valued. If you have been carrying around many of the same beliefs throughout your life then these are old beliefs. These old beliefs may not be potentially beneficial presently, however without being aware of them or something occurring, they may never change.

This is the benefits and purpose for many diseases, just to bring your attention to beliefs that do need to change. Since beliefs are only thoughts, you always have the ability to change what you are choosing to think, however it takes being aware of what you are choosing to think to make the changes. This may sound simple but for most individuals it's more challenging then it appears because old beliefs have had great amounts of powerful energy stored in them. So at first it does take quite a bit of practicing on a daily basis. Just as any practicing takes time at first and after a few weeks the new way becomes just as natural and into a habit as the old way of thinking.

Attitudes are a result of beliefs and you will find through your healing process that your attitudes about many things will change. That will also be great feedback for you too.

Feedback of the New Changes

Feedback is a great tool to noticing changes from the way you reacted before the disease and then after. By taking notice of the differences in the way you react to same situations will show you your feedback. For an example something that continuously irritated you for a long time will create a body rash. Or it may create throat problems and if the belief, which is the thoughts you are choosing probably without you even realizing that you had the choice to choose different thoughts. This is where the feedback and awareness is so important. Before understanding this knowledge of information you may have believed that you did not have a choice in choosing thoughts. Now you become to realize that you always have a choice, in the past it may have appeared you didn't but now you become to see it through awareness. This allows you the opportunity to now choose better thoughts about everything in general. By doing this you will find that all of your old reactions change to new ways to respond without so much negativity. Something that irritated you in the past would no longer trigger that old belief when it is changed. The new way to responding is less stressful on your body while simultaneously your body cells are picking up the new sensations of data of information too. The feelings of peace results in harmonious body cells, the body stays relaxed instead of up tight as in the past.

Remember all illness and disease or pain is a signal and creation of disharmony that the cells picked up in the messaging to respond to create the body to be. This is so empowering to know and can continue to remind you if this is new information for you.

Now knowing that beliefs are just thoughts that have been valued that sustained itself which created a belief system from those valued thoughts. How do you create a new beneficial thought? By choosing better feeling thoughts and doing this consistently whenever you notice old thoughts surfacing, insert the new thoughts so the responding will be different and of the best potential for your health.

A belief is just a thought you thought about long enough and thoughts you have carried through your life. Choosing better thoughts creates better feelings and is how you change a belief.

In the affirmations chapter there is a list of new thoughts that you can use to replace the old disempowering ones whenever they surface. This is a great way to guide you in changing your thoughts. When the new thoughts becomes natural and habitual just as the old way of thinking was originally then you know you have changed beliefs, all because you are now responding differently then in your past.

When you naturally respond differently then you did in the past it is powerful feedback that shows you that you have changed and so will your body too.

Power of Experimenting and Experiencing

No matter how many people tell you their own successes with healing the most powerful will be when you experience it for yourself. Other people's experiences can only guide you in the direction as inspiration to experiencing healing for yourself.

Dream State Realization

Have you awakened from a dream where in the dream you were running or being chased or doing something exertive? When you awakened from the dream you were literally sweating? Or you awoke with a big smile on your face or even laughing of something you were dreaming about? Well this can be the first realization that thoughts and emotions are affecting your body without any physical touching.

One ... Experiment and Experience

Try this right now

Bring yourself to a relaxed state by focusing your thoughts to one thing that is seeing one word that creates a feeling of a relaxed state. It's best to pick a word that triggers the best feelings for you. This may take a bit if you are not familiar with keeping your focus on one thing. Once you are in that relaxed state which should take a few minutes, even if thoughts are still racing, close your eyes and see and feel yourself biting into a sour lemon. Stay with it for awhile really imagining your hand bringing the lemon to your mouth and biting into the sour lemon and your taste buds tasting it. Keep going with the image until you can taste it until you mouth puckers from the sour taste. Have you experienced it?

This is one proof that shows you how powerful our imagination is without a real physical thing but our own mind of focusing thought and emotional feelings. One thought with imagining stirs your emotions into feelings that affect your senses and body. This is directing and steering deliberately your focusing of thought where you put your thoughts into one attention.

Two ... Experiment and Experience

Doing the same thing as the first experiment, bring yourself to a relaxed state and focus on your baby finger on your right side of your hand. Focus on your baby finger and put your full attention on your baby finger and imagine feeling tingling sensations. Don't give up if you have not felt the tingling, keep focusing until you feel it. This is important to do the focusing and not give up until you feel it. If you give up all that means is your beliefs are still so stubborn and staying with it until you feel it is a powerful benefit in so many ways of continued self healing.

What you have done with the lemon imagining and the baby finger imagining is the experiment that creates your own self to experience how powerful your thoughts steered into one focus spot in your body and how it really affects the area. This is the same thing you do for any illness or disease and do not give up until your imagining is removed of all doubt and you only feel the harmony and healed states in your body.

You can start out with something small as a cold or sinus infections and experiment with imagining it healed repetitiously. Every time the cold or sinus infections pops in your mind, insert the imagining of how it feels not to have the cold or sinus infection, even if it's a few minutes and then let it go. Continue to do the imagining until it becomes to feel natural with no longer having any doubts pop in to interrupt the magnificent focus you are putting your attention of thoughts and feelings into. You will eventually experience the cold or sinuses disappearing.

Eventually you will be able to do this for better eyesight. Stare at the page in a book that is blurry and focus your attention not on how blurry the words are but how clear they are becoming and magnified right before your own eyes. I have done this and confirm that it works, it's so amazing and great proof of how our own thoughts are really creating how our body is responding. You can do this for anything that you have created that has become out of harmony, pain, discomfort. Once you have a few experiences from experimenting, that will be all the powerful proof you need to continue all healing.

You will find there will be less to heal in the future because you become so aware from the experiments you do for yourself and the powerful experiences you have which creates more and more harmony in your body. This also means you have created a neuronet of wired memories in your brain and body cells that becomes on command through your thoughts and feelings of how easily you can heal yourself. Remind yourself often that it is YOU WHO IS THE ONE WHO IS COMMANDING YOUR BODY.

Reversing the Process of Thinking

All you are doing is reversing what you have been doing all along. Created disease or any body discomfort or unaltered body condition is a result from going with the focus of the pain, or the blurring of eyesight or the discomfort or the thoughts of more worsening of the disease. When you feel pain in the past you went with it, your focus of attention was on thoughts of how it hurts that continued it to worsen. You were probably unaware that you were even doing it and this is the reason that SELF AWARENESS is so important in knowing how you are choosing to think, not only in healing but in everything in your life.

Remember if you have not experienced any of these experiments, do not give up until you do, this is the most powerful proof you need to get you going and the trust that develops for self healing. The more you experience your successes in the imagining, the more proof you have that creates inspiration and more proof of bigger and bigger things that may still seem doubtful in your belief system. The more you do it, the more the doubt will disappear and on to greater and greater experiences.

You can use these 2 pages to write out a list of what you are working on. As a reminder and even jot down your experiences as you progress. Or keep a journal in the beginning so you can look back on it.

Chapter Seven

Elimination Reveals the Power Source of Now

Thought is Energy
What You Think is what Matters

This may be the most important knowledge that will eliminate everything so that you can know where the power has always been and where it will always be. Everything else is only a medium we use as an in between. When we get to the real source of power you will find, as I have experienced that we then eliminate everything and work from our most powerful source that is the power of now, the present moment.

Mediums I am referring to are things as medications, pills, lucky charms or things we attach thoughts that create the beliefs so that objects then contain lucky energy. Foods, herbal or health food, any liquids we drink and the list can contain anything that is an object or physical thing. Everything that is a physical object is really only a medium that we use to connect a powerful energy through our thoughts about it that gives it any power. We can see evidence in this everywhere once we start to expand our focus with awareness as we observe. Every object can be uniquely defined for everyone unless mass conditioning has already been established and has become a belief system.

Red Wine

As an example let us use red wine. Since it has become in the public media that research has evidence that drinking red wine is healthy for us. Red wine contains anti oxidant proteins that are beneficial for our many organs of our body. Before that became public knowledge, many considered red wine to be just another alcoholic beverage. Unless of course it was an already established belief you already had before hearing the media announcement. I adapted that belief from my younger age as my grandparents believed that red wine was good for them. A belief they carried on from Europe, being they were Italian heritage. So it was an already established belief for myself, I grew up with that belief and carried it throughout my life. Even though I would get headaches from wine if I drank more then two glasses. But then I realized that was only another belief I had created somewhere along the time line. I knew that beliefs can also be changed if I put some work into changing it. Or have less resistance by only having one or two glasses of wine.

For the individuals who had a belief that red wine was just another alcoholic beverage and upon hearing about the new research, they allowed the new information to change their belief instantly. For most individuals it goes unnoticed how their beliefs become changed. This is how easily we can be conditioned about everything if we are not aware of the knowledge about our body, brain and the nature of how reality works. When we do become aware, we can actually choose consciously what we want to believe or not believe. That's the magnificence of the power of awareness and the power of the present moment of NOW and this knowledge of information can go unnoticed for many individuals that are not self aware.

Nothing has Any Power over You

So whether it is wine, pills, herbal teas, or even another individual, it is all the same. Nothing has any power over you in itself, the power is always in your own self. In awareness you can choose to use anything as the medium to be powerful, at least this way you are controlling what you are choosing. You still know the power is in yourself first and you are using the powerful moment of NOW.

Though it may take some practice and experimenting for yourself to see the evidence of what I am explaining, if you do, you will also see all the evidence come to light.

Medication

Another example is medication. The majority of the populations believe that medication is helpful in healing, yet it never heals, it only lessens the pain of the symptoms, but for other individuals they may believe the opposite.

If an individual has given enough valued thought to all medication being poisonous to their body, that's exactly the command the body would react in creating the body's response to be created. So the belief that's created is that medication is toxic and the person may become very sick from medication. Yet for another person who believe medication is good then the belief creates the opposite, makes them feel better.

It has nothing to do with the pill or medication itself, it is the individual's belief that gives the effect always. It's just most of the population has been conditioned to believe that pills or medication and doctors advice is the best thing one can do. Yet for an individual who does not believe that belief it would create an opposite reaction. This is the power of belief and the power that is within each of us. But it's the knowledge of information concerning how our body and body system and cells and brain work. How the nature of reality works.

This knowledge is empowering because it brings you right back to the powerful source of it all. Though it may take a bit for your beliefs to change to accept this new knowledge, it is worth whatever you must go through to establish the new beliefs.

The new beliefs will form and support the new you through the healing process. By eliminating all mediums that we in our past gave our power to is an evolving expanding experience. Even as you may go through some shaking stages, as I have through the trusting process, it has all been so worth it.

The Placebo Affect

The placebo affect is so encouraging because massive research through experiments and what the results have shown. Researchers gave individuals a sugar pill when they are told they were getting medication that would relieve pain, while they gave another group of individuals the real medication. The results were profound because the individuals who were given the sugar pills were relieved of pain just as the individuals who were given the real medication. This proved to show that it has nothing to do with the pills and what they contained and had everything to do with the suggestions and their beliefs. The individuals who took the sugar pills believed the placebo would work because they believed it was real medication, it had nothing to do with the pills at all. There are so many experiences you can read about just by searching the internet on placebo affects. And you should because the more you read about these experiments and the proof of the power of suggestions and beliefs create more powerful memories. Especially if you have stubborn beliefs, reading about these types of experiences become a catalyst in creating the powerful changes in you to support the new revelations.

I know if you are really committed and serious about healing yourself then you will search everything you need to find to support the new you. When you keep your focus on healing you will be amazed how everything you need to know will come to you through synchronicity.

Our Body has a Language

You will find eventually you no longer need any medium to tell you what's wrong or right with your body, you will find that your body does a great job in communicating to you all the time.

How much better could it get, Your body has a language that communicates to you what is going on and all you have to do is listen in the language it's communicating in. This has always been going on from your body to you, the only difference is that you didn't know how to listen to what your body was trying to tell you. You needed a medium for the only reason being because you were not taught that the body has a language. The language of our body's communication is through pain or no pain. How we feel is how it communicates to us. So now you can decipher the communication yourself, the more you do it, the better you also become at it.

Chapter Eight

Loving Your Disease
Or
Pain

Do you think you can love your disease or pain?

I know at first this may sound uncomfortable or absurd and challenging to do, however it is a very powerful step in healing and change.

Usually whenever you are in pain or find out you have a disease, your first reaction is fear. Fear seems to be a normal reaction, mostly for the reason of feeling as if you have no control, remember that is victim mentality thinking? It is a result of your belief that you do not have power over your disease from not trusting yourself yet. Taking the fear feeling by transforming fear thoughts to love thoughts will change your feeling and the way you continue to perceive it now in the powerful present moment.

Loving your disease or pain with the knowledge that you have read in the previous chapters. Loving your disease or pain for what it is showing you of what you did not know previously, but are now learning about yourself and your beliefs. And also for all it will teach you along the way to your healing.

Loving it because it is a part of you, your body, it is you, so loving it is so important and to love without conditions or judgments. This transforms all fear thoughts that are energy into love thoughts of energy. Love energy is accepting and allowing the process of healing to continue, even when you still have days that the pain or disease still shows up. And it will until you have responded differently then in your past, that is when you will know you really have changed. By continuing to love your body and its disease and what it is communicating to you, is adding more love by listening to your body's language. Paying attention to your body's communication is loving it.

Think of your body as a close friend of yours. If your friend is verbally conversing with you about a problem they are having, would you ignore them? Most probably you would listen with compassionate and try to soothe them as best you can. This is the same way with your body, when you react with fear and then transform the energy to love thoughts would be the same as with your listening to your friend. You would not scream at your friend with anger and fear, as you know that would upset them more. Instead you would listen and try to help. This is the same way to respond with your body and the disease or pain as it is communicating to you. Responding by loving it, is accepting it and continuing to love it to bring it to a quicker healing.

Love will always bring healing quicker and fear will always create it to become in more pain, increasing the disease to worsen.

Before I became knowledgeable about self healing, whatever I experienced as pain, be it a migraine, or flu, cold, ear ache, vertigo, chest pain, sinuses, back aches, heart problems and more, I reacted in fear too. Each time I worked my own self healing I realized I was creating more memories to be created that I would be able to retrieve in the future. These new memories create the trust we need to continue self healing. There were stages I went through that I would question and have doubts at first, so it does take practice and continuing so that trusting yourself becomes easier and natural. All doubt is only retrieved from the old beliefs, and I would remind myself many times of this information until it did become natural and the new way with self healing.

So nothing is too big or incurable for you when you come to realize and know that it was you all along that have created the pain or disease to begin with. That gives you power back in the powerful present moment, now just from knowing this wisdom from your own experiences along the healing process.

How long you stay in fear before you finally choose to consciously transform the fear to love is always up to you. Remembering that the fear is only a habit from the old beliefs. Transform fear to love so that you will then have new beliefs to support the new healed you.

Chapter Nine

Self
Healing
Stages

For some individual they do not go through self healing stages at all. This is referred to as miraculous and instantaneous healings. We find deeper revelations that allow the instant healings to occur which is actually a belief so strong, pure and unaltered that creates any disease to be instantly healed. There is staggering amounts of evidence presently to support this amazing instant healing. Yet for many individuals they do not experience instant healing because they still have beliefs that dictate and create healings to take time. For these individuals, myself included in my past of the beliefs that contains thoughts that dictate that it takes time to go through these stages. It's a belief commanding us to think we have to go through stages and if that's what it takes we can use these stages to be beneficial to our evolving growth.

We also will find as we go through our stages of healing it's beneficial because the time it takes will have many great learning experiences along the way. So just as in everything when we allow opportunity of growth that will evolve us to learn unconditional love to be embedded in our experiences of any disease, we will also learn and grow a great deal from these experiences.

Stage One –
Finding out You have a disease

You find out you have a disease, usually it is by medical authorities. If we do not go to a doctor, as I do not, then I can only go by what I feel of my body's communication. I will not even know if something I am going through is a disease of some sort. However for the majority of people a disease is confirmed by the medical field.

Stage Two –
Accepting the disease

The time gap of denial into acceptance may take the path of fear until it reaches a hopeful stage. This stage is unique with every individual on the length of time that individuals go in and out of this stage. Some longer then others. For some they may even die with the disease and never have taken their power back. But if you continue to read and take the empowering journey of self healing then you continue to the next stages.

Stage Three –
Realizing you have power to change

In this stage you come to the realization that you have the power to change the disease. There are many individuals who use this stage differently then accepting that they are powerful beings, if they leave it in the hands of a more powerful healer. Examples of an actual healer healing them, or God or any religion or cultural worship. For myself and throughout this book I am referring to our own self as having the power because since we are created in the image of The Creator. And genetically we do have encoded within us of an Infinite Creator, then for me, that is enough to know it's inherit within us already. Then we harness the power by realizing this disease created was generated and progressed by what we have chosen to think into emotions to feel that created the disease for our own urgings to know the power we have within. If an individual is born with a disease then I believe it's for a purposeful infinite reason too, carried on from another lifetime. They can use the same knowledge throughout this book, to use the disease as an opportunity to learn, grow and evolve as a result.

Stage Four –
Using the power of Imagination to create the change into healing

Using the power of your imagination to change your directions on how and what you think about so that your body can reflect the creation of the changes.

Stage Five –
Sustaining the Power of Already Healed

Though this is last in the list it is actually the most important and powerful because without this stage our disease will continue to resurface. This is what occurs if a person goes to a healer and is healed but the disease comes back because the individual has not changed completely. This is the reason it is so powerful to heal yourself, you go through the stages you need to go through and never have to refer to another person again.

It takes imagining long enough that you see and feel the disease or whatever it is you are healing to be already healed. Not in the process of already being healed because that is more waiting time.

Whenever you imagine make sure you are imagining yourself as it would feel if you were healed. See and feel exactly how it would feel if you no longer had the pain, had the disease or whatever it is you have unconsciously or consciously created as a disharmony in your body.

Again this is such an important step that if any doubts surface you just love them and let them go, in other words delete them immediately and insert the already healed again image. Create the imaging as a video in your mind. This way you are adding in the feelings in motion until it becomes so natural and so automatic that you no longer even have to think about doing it, it becomes automatic and is now how you think.

Chapter Ten

States of Being

Already Healed
is a
Love State

Our state of being is so powerful that whatever state of being we are in is exactly what is creating our reality and our body simultaneously. Our state of being is whatever we are thinking that becomes our gathered emotions that we then experiences as our feelings.

If we are in a state of being anxious about something then we are generating from fear thoughts that swirl the gathering of fear emotions that generate how we then are feeling. The feeling is always the end result from what we have given our attention of thoughts to. So we are in a state of being of fear, experiencing anxious nervous feelings and our body is always paying attention to our thoughts and state of being even when we are not aware. It's working and functioning and creating all the time.

The state of being is how you are feeling right now. Then how you feel in the next moment, then the next and then next hour and so on. However you are feeling is what your STATE OF BEING is from a result of your thinking.

Being aware as much as we possibly can especially in the beginning stages of choosing new thoughts is essential. If we do not keep ourselves aware in the beginning it's too easy to fall back to the old patterns and beliefs of thoughts as in the past that created the disease originally.

When we take a look at the opposite direction of fear and observe our state of being in love, we then notice a completely different state of being. When we are excited about something, we can hardly keep ourselves grounded. We feel so lifted as a result of the excitement we are reveling in. This is a state of being that is generating joy, fun, laughter, love, we can not only see and feel the difference, and we know the differences of the two comparisons.

One of a state of being in fear, the other experience of a state of being in love with someone or something and it should always start with being in love with our self first and with no judgments or conditions.

Try this right Now

Think of something that scares you, maybe it's a big unpaid bill, or something that you are worried about, just think about something that puts you in an anxious and fearful mood or state of being. Have you done it? Good! You know how that fear feels as your state of being.

Now do this, think of something or someone that creates feelings of such joy, excitement or love. Think about it for awhile, really immerse yourself in the thoughts and feelings of what really stirs your emotions of love, excitement, joy. Have you done it? Good!

Now notice the difference of how you felt in the fearful state of being compared to the loving state of being. Oh I know this is simple stuff but remember the most simple stuff can go unnoticed. Just realize that you experienced 2 different states of being.

One tensed your body, this is the disharmony state of being. The other love state of being relaxed and lifted the body. Now realize that really if we make it really simple that we can just realize that there is **fear** and **love** and anything else that falls into those 2 categories are only extensions, expansions of the two energies.

So **state of being** are experiences we are in all the time depending on what we are thinking about that will be generating how we are feeling. Either in the fear category list or the love category list and expands in either direction the longer we keep ourselves in the state of that particular being.

State of Being Already Healed is the Love State of Being

To be in a state of being as already healed may take some practice if you are not already familiar with imagining or visualizing your desires in advance. It seems to be how the universe and creation of the nature of reality works. And healing works the same way.

Whatever state of being we are in is what is creating our body cells to create. So the most potential state of being to be is to allow healing to be created by being in a state of being already healed and that is a love state. This state of being already healed gathers its momentum of thoughts and emotions into feelings into a natural expectation that allows the healing to be created.

How do you be in a state of being already healed? By continuously keeping your thoughts and feelings and imaginings on already healed. What would it feel like to be already healed? What would you be thinking of if you were already healed? Perpetually imagining and feeling as if you were already healed every time the disease thought pops up, will continue the healing process. And that in itself is loving your self and loving every experience you are creating and going through with no conditions or judgments. Just because you really were created out of Infinite Love of an Infinite Creator. Accepting this wisdom is the catalyst for all healing in every area of your life because genuinely loving yourself with your heart and soul is the ultimate vibration to always be in. It heals anything and everything and is the most precious secret to know.

Chapter Eleven

The New You
With
Great Experience

You will notice that this new road of thoughts will transform your perception too. You may be sitting at the same window while drinking your coffee, but the coffee taste better even though it's the same coffee maker, the same coffee brand. The same window you always look out every morning, you notice something has changed.

It sure has, **you have changed**. You are appreciating the moment, you are responding with love, a very high vibration energy of frequency. Your body has already picked up on the new changes and messages and now you are experiencing the results. The coffee tastes better then ever, the scene outside the same window is more alive and brighter. Something that previously would have stressed you out, now does not even bother you. You just smile in awe of it all and are so enlightened to have gone through all that you went through to experience this change.

Now you get excited for the next sign post that bothers you and you again get to work on the new direction again. You are amazed how it has become exciting instead of in the past when things were dreaded. Slowly but surely each day becomes renewed of this awe and passionate love that you welcome all new sign posts as your opportunity to keep changing directions. The new unwinding, unfolding journey has started and is progressing and you are just loving it all.

Before you even realize it, your body has less and less pain, till eventually there is no pain. Days upon days or it could take weeks or months have gone by and no more pain. If you are diligently consistent on this new chosen path you will find that medical tests have changed. Results of your illness or disease you had is either dissolving or completely disappeared. If the disease continues to reappear then it will always be a sign of feedback to get your attention to show you what has been going on. A sign to change direction again with your thoughts and verbal conversations.

You notice you are no longer urged to turn the news on, you no longer want to talk about depressing things. You feel the differences so sensitively now because you really have become more sensitized through your powerful awareness. You actually say bring it on!

When another person starts talking depressing things then you enjoy transforming the conversation to more uplifting things and then you either notice that they other all of a sudden says, "I gotta go" and conversation has ended. The reason being some individuals rather have misery being a comforter, meaning the belief, "misery likes company" well for you, you don't anymore. You realize the difference and what a difference it literally makes in your body and your life. You have now become a love or bliss transformer and you love it so much that nothing is going to alter you from it. You will notice that more then ever others you talk to don't hang up and not want to stop talking, instead you begin to notice when you are transforming a negative conversation into a positive one that the other starts to join in. The more you notice this experience, you can know absolutely you have really changed because your environment is mirroring to show you the proof.

You will notice you'd rather go for a walk than sit in front of the television and watch a show. You hear nature's calling, those chirping birds urging you on, gee's you wonder why you didn't notice that before? It's because you really have changed and what an exuberant celebration it is. You will notice more and more changes that are exhilarating and exciting, and this love vibrational journey will passionately keep urging you on. How could it not when it feels so good and changes so much.

It does not take long of basking in the new you for awhile to be able to notice the contrast of the new you of love to the old you of pain out of fear. This contrast is another celebration because it will become easier to notice and continue to keep switching to the new loving you more often. Until you find the old you is experienced less and less and the new you becomes to take over easier then ever. Then you know you are on the way to a complete and lasting desirous change.

You realize it was worth everything you went through and eventually everything really is blissful no matter what is going on and you notice less chaos then ever before. You are now on the blissful journey, what many refer to as heaven on earth.

Chapter Twelve

Reminiscing
With
Appreciation Consistently

Being in a state of thankfulness is appreciating your disease, pain or disharmony. If it was not for the pain or disease, you may not have changed.

Change seems to come about for many through experiences that push them into it. Many die when diseases become extreme or to the point that it seems it could never be cured or healed, in other words hopeless. It's important to remember that nothing is hopeless or impossible except for the beliefs that dictate that to be the truth and by now you know that a belief is only a thought you kept thinking and you have the power to change any belief you no longer want.

Anything is possible and more then ever on our planet presently people are healing themselves all the time. So we need to remove impossible out of our belief system all together. So that we can allow our bodies to perform as they naturally have the ability to do. Heal itself.

Once all of this information is understood from your own experiences that you use as your proven feedback, it will be easy and simple to comprehend that everything is possible. In this state of mind which is the state of being of love and appreciation goes hand in hand. You are gratefully thankful for your disease and all that you went through that has created the experience that you have evolved. You have surpassed hopelessness into empowerment from your own experiences, this now is your own wisdom. You appreciate not only your disease or pain, you appreciate many other things that in the past you did not appreciate.

As you reminisce of all your experiences of the past in the present, your realization is illuminated into thankfulness for it all. That is growth that is expanding your consciousness and evolving into new wisdom for yourself. You are also thankful with appreciation that you can now share your experiences with others to help them on their healing journey. If I can do it, you can do it and when you do it any other can too. It's the new evolution that is going on presently on our planet. You are now a part of that evolution and you become so appreciative of it.

You reminisce of the past memories in elation of the changes you went through. You clearly see how the old beliefs of thoughts actually created the disease or pain and all of this appreciation continuously flows into everything, when you allow it to.

To be able to appreciate the disease or pain and to appreciate the difference now of having no pain or disease.

Appreciation becomes a natural habit compared to the old beliefs of the past. You will find it's easy to find things to appreciate during and after your healing. It does become a new way of living and your body responds harmonious continuously when you sustain everything in an appreciative ways that really does lead to bliss.

Chapter Thirteen

Releasing Built up Toxins

Releasing toxins from your body is essential to healing because releasing toxins is what healing is all about.

What is a toxin?
Anything that is out of harmony of your natural process of peace, relaxed state, positive, good feelings. So this clearly shows us that anything that we react with fear that extends into the energy of anger, frustration, hate, confusing, blame creates feelings of disharmony. This is

also the opposite of genuine unconditional love. If you are in the disharmony state for too long, toxins are building in your body. This reacting in disharmony is an end result of your beliefs. Whatever you believe about anything that you judge as not good is creating toxins, which is the disharmony of your body cells. Negative fear thoughts are toxic and actually creates the toxicity in our body that creates emotional blockages.

As an example, you know those days where the day is going on so good and then something seems to appear to happen and then your day takes a turn for the worse. This has a two fold learning experience when this occurs, firstly the day only turned to the worst because of your belief. Secondly that turning point is when the toxins build up and if you are not aware it can build up for months and years. This is the power of awareness, you will read more about this in the next chapter. The more self aware we become, the less toxins we will be building up in our body because we know that we are the one who is building the toxins in the first place. It is extremely helpful to remind yourself that it will always be the way you react to everything that will change the way the body reproduces toxins or no toxins. Eventually if you continue to be aware and react differently about everything that you reacted negatively in the past, fear energy and respond positively of the love energy, you will see the changes. You will notice fewer toxins which means you will notice you are less sick.

Ways of Releasing Toxins

These built up toxins must be released, and many times you will find your body will release it naturally just by getting in a better mood. Now you can be aware of how your body is releasing its toxins and do it before any diseases get a chance to build up before you body becomes extremely toxic. Let's take a look at ways our body releases toxins.

Crying is a powerful release

Anytime we cry we are releasing toxins from our body. Toxins build up as a result of staying in our past too long, via thoughts, verbally conversing as we do when we talk about the past. Also toxins build up if we hold too much in without allowing the flow in some way to release.

You know those days you have when it seems just out of the blue you start to cry, whether it's because of a commercial or whatever triggered the tears, you just did not expect it. Well that is a sure sign of build up toxins that may have taken months or years before it finally came to a release. I know for myself I noticed in hindsight that I didn't cry for years, then when crying started to release it became more often then in my past.

The body has built up too many toxic negative chemicals and then naturally releases it. As I recall up to the years before the release of crying that I was sick a lot too. If there is no release there is build up and if we continue to hold back any release then we create disease and illnesses. So when the sporadic tearful crying comes on, go with it and let it all out and know you are releasing built up toxic past issues of emotions.

Anyway that you can find that is the beneficial way to cry to release the built up toxins. It may be reading a book, or watching a movie, or a commercial, or something that another has said to you. When you allow yourself to be creative, you will surely surprise yourself of the many ways that you can release built up toxins. Eventually it will become natural to be more aware of your thoughts during your day and you will find less toxins built up to release.

We all know how much better we feel after a good cry or a good sleep and it's all a result of the release. I find now that I cry so easily and all it means is the big blockages I had in the past are now free flowing. When this occurs we have become sensitive and that is such a great sign. No longer are we blocked, like a dam that prevents flow, clogs arteries, and you thought it was the food that clogged blood flow? Remember it's always about what we think about what we eat that gives what we eat the power in our body to create anything to be.

Sleep is a powerful release

Sleep is a powerful release because when we sleep our body regenerates itself while we are busy in another dimensional reality. In that other dimensional reality we are working out what needs to be worked out that we didn't work out during our awake time. If you dream of a fight then it's releasing what was building up in you that you didn't deal with previously. You dreams can tell you a lot about your waking reality. Though it is passed on in the illusion that when we sleep and dream, we are just dreaming. When we probe deeper behind the illusion, we can see clearly what is really going on.

Anything you have not resolved in your waking time will be what you work out in your dreams. There may be filtered meanings when you awake in recalling your dreams. As an example, in your dreams you may have been fighting a dragon. Deciphering the meanings to align with what is going on in your waking life will make more sense out of it all. The dragon may represent a person you are having a difficult time with in your waking dimension of life. However even though you are working it out in your dream reality, if you continue to react the same way continuously with the appearing difficult person, you will continue to dream this way too. Because it will be working out the waking reality in the dream reality continuously. This is the importance of working as much as we can in awareness in our waking reality. Then you will recall dreams that are more blissful and enjoyable too. Well unless of course you associate fighting with pleasure then that is another scenario of belief to deal with and work out.

So dreaming is a natural release of built up toxins of our waking reality. This is the reason that when things become too overwhelming to the point of exhausting you, it's best to have a nap, sleep to reenergize your body and allow your dreams to work it out. Even if you do not recall your dreams, you are always dreaming when you sleep. The recollection of the dream is only farther away in your memories to recall, but you always dream when you sleep. You have to because you are really experiencing another dimension for awhile.

Journaling is a powerful release

Journaling is very therapeutic way of releasing any built up emotions that are a result of negative thoughts we have been lingering in too long. Journaling is similar to writing in a diary, except a diary is what we write about our experiences and desires as they happen. In journaling we write not only of the experiences we go through but also add in any things we want to change and our awareness and future desires.

One day of journaling can fill pages of a note book. You may start to journal about what is bothering you, and then you progress through the release while writing what is bothering you and then awareness comes through simultaneously. I found in the beginning as I continue to journal any past stuff of what was bothering me I then began writing what I have learned from it all. Then I continue to write the changes I will make and before I realize it I was then writing in a positive loving way.

Sometime crying occurs through the journaling as it naturally brings on the triggering of releases of build up. Always by the end of my journaling I feel so much better and more optimistic. It transforms all negativity into positive, stress to bliss, doubt to hope, fear to love, knowing to elation and back to empowerment. Whether you are writing in a journal or maybe writing a fictional story, it will still be a process of releasing anything built up.

Video is a powerful release

You can speak freely using your video camera to record yourself as you speak to release what you have suppressed. Just speaking about what is bothering you and keep talking until you transform the negative to the positive. I did this years ago. Later when I listened to the recordings it illuminated to show me how much I had grown through the evolving stages.

Recording your release decreases having to talk about it throughout the day to others. When we do that we are then lingering in the negativity and adding more to it by conversing with another or others about what is bothering us. This gives more powerful energy to stir up more negativity and judgment energies. When you release by speaking verbally out loud into a recorder device you will find you easily and naturally release and then when you speak to others it will be about positive things. Is it not better to perpetuate the positive energy then the negative? Whether we are thinking about something or speaking about it, speaking will be more powerful because you are adding verbalized voice that is a stronger energy force as usually emotions become entangled into the verbal too.

Animals are a powerful release

I know many of us already do this consistently if we have pets. If we do not have pets we may find when we are out in nature we may just converse, thinking out loud or think as we observe birds or a tree. Animals usually love without any conditions and instantly forgive. It seems to be a natural built in quality for most animals. If some domesticated animals seen to have a tainted personality when they are bothered, it's a mixture of the pet and the pet owner's a mirror reflective perceptional energies. Even though wild animals must kill to survive to eat, they also have an unconditional gene.

The majority of animals seem to be very therapeutic for us when we confide in them, even though they are just there unconditionally and loving. Whether it is just quietly stroking their fur while we think whatever is bothering us long enough to find some peace about it. Our animals sit there enjoying our interactions. Some of us may talk to our animals as if they really are human beings and of course for the one's that do talk to them, we do know they also understand what we are communicating.

When you allow yourself to be creative, you will surely surprise yourself on the many way that you can release built up toxins. Eventually it will become natural to be more aware of your thoughts during your day and you will find less toxins built up to release.

Chapter Fourteen

The Power
of
Self Awareness

In the last chapter and throughout this book I mention about self awareness because it is the most powerful part of any healing. It takes being self aware to actually create the progression of self healing. Without self awareness we will only be living life from old automatic programming of beliefs and that is what creates all disease. Other than instantaneous healing which is instantaneous awareness.

To be self aware means that you are noticing as much as humanly possible throughout the day of the thoughts you are choosing that is creating how and what you are talking about to others. And your own self talk that you say or think to yourself and how you react about everything and everyone.

Being self aware is constantly keeping your attention on You and every time you notice it is not on you, you bring your attention back to you. In the old beliefs is was considered to be conceited to love yourself or to have your attention on yourself but that is just another false conditioning belief. The truth is the exact opposite of that old belief.

Self awareness is not about any vanity, it is all about knowing yourself and how empowering it becomes for you and your life and all others you ever interact with too. Without self awareness we would not know what we believe and what we believe creates everything in our lives.

You can notice it in everything, how can one person eat the same thing as another and yet each individual will have a different affect? Just take a look at diseases, how can one person smoke and another who took extreme care of themselves without smoking and eating healthy and exercising, yet they become sick with cancer and the other does not? This is all proof and a result of individual's belief systems.

Let us again remind ourselves what a belief is. A belief is just a thought you thought about long enough or carried from past conditioning throughout your life. Either way it is a belief, the way to change a belief is to think different thoughts long enough until the old belief no longer has any triggered energy to react. However it will always take being self aware to even realize that you believe a certain way about certain things or experiences to then have the power to change the beliefs. Actually what we are really doing is creating new beliefs to override the old ones. We can never destroy the memories of old beliefs but when we override them with newer potentially better thoughts with feelings we create new memories that will be triggered eventually automatically as the old belief worked.

Chapter Fifteen

Self Healing and Love

Love is so important for self healing because without it you will not heal. All disease is a result from not loving yourself originally, so to bring your body's natural harmony back into alignment it really all starts with love.

Think about it, the only reason that you became diseased is because you fell out of love with yourself. You allowed probably without noticing which means not being self aware which also means subconsciously you entertained too many thoughts of judgments on yourself and on others and situations.

We all have done it because it seems to be human nature to judge and the biggest part in evolution to transform all the judging into acceptance, peace and love. It's the awareness that judging especially in any negative way is creating disharmony not only in our bodies but also in the creation of experiences in our lives too. Timing of anything in out of synch or just not the way you wanted it, things just do not seem to turn out the way you wanted. When you observe through awareness you will then be able to notice many of these types of out of alignment, out of synchronicity that have manifested in your life. This is the power of self awareness.

When you come to realize and know that all disease starts with a separation from love you will then also realize it takes returning to love for healing to occur.

When you begin your self healing or even your curiosity about self healing that is the beginning of you returning to love, whether you were aware of it or not, that is what is occurring. You are caring enough about yourself to not want anymore pain or disease that you become inspired to know more about what is happening in your body. You also come to a point that you will do whatever it takes to heal it too. That is all returning to loving and caring about yourself first, falling in love with you that you care that much about you now.

Loving Yourself First

We have all heard the statement that we can never love another if we do not love our self first and I used to wonder about that statement because I have loved others even when I did not think I loved myself first. I came to realize that I was only loving others to the **degree that I loved myself.**

Everything is always to the degree of the reflection of ourselves that we see externally in our environment.

It became very clear for me as I observed more and more of how I loved others when I observed with self awareness. I found that sure I was loving others but only to the degree and reflection of my own self love. So in other words when I loved myself but with still lots of judgments, I was also loving others with judgments. Many times the judgments would not surface until someone did something that I did not agree with or that I did not like. By the reflection of the experiences I realized how I was judging myself first and then the love reflection was mirrored out of the other.

The more that I learned and experimented with self love through self awareness, the more that I became aware of the kind of love I had for myself that continued to reflect outward. This is so powerful because when we come to this stage we then perceive everything and everyone in our own reflection and it is also when we create the most potential growth in our self too.

Another powerful awareness was my ability to change many things that I was judging but did not realize it until I worked consistently on being self aware of how I loved myself.

When another did something I did not like, I immediately took it as a sign to turn my attention back to me and ask myself, what is it that creates these beliefs of judging another in certain ways that I was judging them? I found it all came back to my beliefs that I had and as I worked on changing my old beliefs I began to notice that the things that I did not like about others became what I learned to accept and allow that created more love. I became excited each time I noticed anything that would surface that I did not like or agree upon in any other. It became a powerful catalyst for learning so much about myself that I did not know when I was projecting my reflective beliefs onto others. It is like a trick that gives us the illusion to believe that others are really the one that is bothering us when it is really our own self of beliefs to begin with. The more I worked on this the more that I became to love myself because I continued to work on acceptance of myself first then I would see it reflected in others.

As a result I was blaming less and less, I became more tolerant that then turned into compassion and empathy. I observed so many negative beliefs that created a filtering of my own beliefs onto others become to dissolve. Eventually the empathy returned to such a loving state that no matter what another one was going through I could stay neutral to have no judgment at all. Realizing that everyone has a bigger reason for whatever they are going through to grow as a result, even if they were not aware of it. Judging became less and less and love became more and more unconditional in all experiences.

The end result of perpetually returning back to love is that negativity transforms to positive through the beginning stages and then both negative and positive transforms to a neutral non judging state of being.

What does that mean then as you go through the transformation of returning to self love first and then observing it in everything you see reflected outward? It means that you have taken every negative and judging situation and used it as an opportunity to use it all as a reflection back to you. You learned more about yourself then you ever knew previously and the negative and positive become transformed into pure unconditional love for yourself first and then everyone and everything and everyone you see and interact with becomes the same, unconditionally loved. You will realize that you can not heal until you love yourself first because if you experience any healing or feeling good for awhile you will not sustain it unless it is changed in your belief system. In other words the disease can reappear at another time in your life and will continue to do so until you get to the root source. And that root source is your own genuine self love first.

Loving Yourself

Loving yourself means that whenever you walk by a mirror you notice that you no longer judge anything about yourself. You love yourself with no conditions or judgments. So in the beginning your first thoughts of judgment may have been judging that you are too overweight or judged your hair or whatever it is about what you seen in the mirror.

In the later stages of working on yourself you walk by a mirror and respond by just smiling at yourself. You no longer notice any imperfections. You realize that all imperfections are just man made judgments of opinions that others have created that so many have accepted without thinking about what they accepted as a belief. Unconditional love is accepting without any conditions, just because you are YOU and alive and aware that you are a Being. You will also know that you are originally and always a Being of Infinite Love.

You will find that the more you love yourself unconditionally, everything takes care of itself. If you are overweight when you love yourself all that extra weight is really old baggage of toxic thoughts that you have held onto for so long, judging thoughts. They really do release in weight physically the more you love yourself with no conditions. It has to because love thoughts are light and uplifting and carry less weight.

You will notice that you start to even see clearer and use your glassed less, this is another symptom of self love. Because in the past you subconsciously did not like what was going on to see closer to you or away from you, depending on which way your eye sight deteriorated. Just as pain becomes less and less or more and more too. Loving yourself without conditions is the most powerful thing you can do, not only for yourself but as you will notice in everyone and thing you experience.

It will become automatic the more you work on loving yourself to see the best in yourself which then allows you to see the best in others, regardless of any situation or experience.

You will come to know as I have that you will always love others in the degree that you love yourself. Doesn't that make it all worth it?

Now if you are not familiar or not sure how to start loving yourself, this next technique will start the process. Continue with the next chapter on affirmations and imagination as it will guide you to the steps that will return yourself to loving yourself. Also check out at the end of the book for extended info and websites. Even if at first it may feel a bit uncomfortable, this is your greatest stage to work through. You must continue and I guarantee if you do you will find that you will become more and more comfortable as you go. You will get to the point that you will wonder how you could have ever not loved yourself because loving yourself is the most powerful, healing natural state of being you will find it to be.

Do this Right Now – Mirror Technique of Feedback of Self Love

You can try this right now and this will show you as feedback so quickly about your own self love. Go to a mirror and look into it and be aware of the first thoughts and feelings that come up for you as you look in the mirror.

Now try this, this is from Louise Hay's teachings, look in the mirror and say to yourself, "I love you!" What thoughts pop up, what feelings come up? If it feels uncomfortable then you can continue this technique during different stages of your progress and you will notice and see the differences from your first time doing this compared to doing it through different stages as you progress in loving yourself. It is powerful feedback.

The last stage is when you can hold up the mirror and love yourself genuinely and feel so good about it with no resistance. That means all resistance has dissolved and the new self love journey is what you are on. And that does change everything literally you will find.

Chapter Sixteen

Self Healing
Affirmations and Imagination

Affirmations

Affirmations are powerful as they are a tool to remind you and keep you on tract with your desire, to heal your disease. You must read them over and over for awhile until they become a natural habit that replaces the old way you used to think and feel and speak. The longer you do read them over, especially when you are in a trance like state, the easier it will record into our subconscious mind. If you are consistent, then within just a few weeks you will start to notice that you will be actually thinking and responding with the affirmations instead of the old way.

Always Affirm and Imagine in the Present

The list I have provided below can be added to or even changed to support your desires for healing. However it is crucial to always create and read your affirmations in the present tense. The same way you do when you visualize or imagine your desires. It is always in the present tense stated or imagined as your desire already manifested or your body as already healed.

The present tense implants the affirming suggestion stronger so it can easily surpass the old subconscious programming that you have been using in the past. When you add feelings and appreciation of being thankful in advance as if you are already healed you will notice quicker healings too.

Think of it this way through this analogy. If you seen a beautiful cloud and wanted to be able to look at it again, which way would be the quickest? To draw a picture of it or just snap a picture with a camera? Well the answer of course is to take a picture that you can then download on your computer or print out and then you could always creatively draw a picture later if you wanted. Since clouds move so quickly you will have to be quick to capture it. This is the similar when you are healing and adding emotional feelings to your thoughts as already healed, it just works faster.

Healing and Healed Affirmations

- My body is a natural rhythm of creation showing me its creation daily. I am in harmony with love, I love myself because I know I was created from the most infinite accepting love.

- Trillions of my body cells are dancing harmoniously responding to all my appreciation, pure love, bliss and joy in my life

- I choose the better thoughts that trigger the better feelings that transforms everything to harmony and bliss

- Before sleep I visualize and choose the thoughts of my healed body. Upon awakening I continue the thoughts of my healed body.

- I am noticing my body feeling better and better

- I realize now it is my thoughts and feelings that have created the disharmony and I notice how quickly choosing the better feeling thoughts makes all the difference in my healing.

- I am in a state of being already healed

- I so easily transform everything to bliss thoughts and feelings and know all the benefits are occurring in my body right now

- I forgive so easily because I know that its never worth altering from my blissful state for no one or no thing

- I easily make peace with everyone and everything

- It's becoming easier and easier to be blissful and peaceful

- I continually use every opportunity to being excited to transforming everything to bliss

- I love the feeling of staying in bliss and experiencing the results I feel so greatly in my body and in all my experiences

Use this Page to Add Your Own Affirmations

Use this Page to Add Your Own Affirmations

Self Healing
and
Imagination

Imagination is the most powerful way to design the blueprint of anything you desire to experience. Using your imagination consciously, deliberately by imagining or visualizing whatever it is you want long enough with intense emotional feelings. Emotions are scattered throughout your body until they are gathered together through our hearts into feelings. Feelings are so powerful because they are the fuel that ignites and runs the imaging to perfection.

Let's use an analogy of a still photograph as our thoughts and a video as our feelings, so we can get a deeper realization of the power of feelings. We can look at a photograph while our imagination gathers thoughts and feelings as we perceive a picture. Though it is a still picture, we gather enough information to bring some aliveness to it. Comparing a video to a photograph, we have a moving picture with sound that stimulates more feelings as a result. If it is a sad picture you feel a little sadness, but if you watch a video of something sad it will evoke more emotions that you will feel. You may even experience crying as a result as empathy becomes triggered. When we compare this analogy of the still picture to a video and our thoughts as the picture and our feelings as a video, you can clearly acknowledge the differences when feelings are added to thoughts.

Imagination Visualizations

You can use this visualization by either just reading through it or record it to listen so that you can close your eyes and relax better. If you record it your focus will be totally present on what you are listening to and guide you along with your focus of thoughts and feelings. You can also change the "you" to "I" do whatever you prefer.

Energy Chakra Centers

In this imagination visualization I use the energy chakra areas. If you are not familiar with your energy chakra areas you can learn more about it from further reading from Martin Brofman's website that is referred to at the end of this book. I also use the counting in breathing of 5 counts of inhale breath, then 7 counts exhale breath as that correlates with our heart spin that will be of the highest breathing potential.

Imagination Visualization

Close your eyes and focus your thoughts and attention on a the beautiful amazing sunset you are now watching as you sit in a rocking chair, rocking back and forth. You are sitting outside as the warm breeze of wind is caressing your skin. You can hear the frogs singing their tunes of rhythmic sounds as they echo through the wind. You are amazed again even though you have seen so many sunsets, everyone is unique and this sunset is radiating its colors of reds, blue's, violet, purplish mixes with pinks transforming together. You feel your body relaxing into the tranquil experience of your vision as the sunset radiates the sky. As you continue in your relaxed state to observe the sunset, feel all the healing colors penetrating through your body, especially any parts of your body that are in pain or discomfort or disease. See and feel the healing colors of the sunset in the sky touch your body and know it is healing it. Gently as the colors soothe through your skin, relaxing you even more.

Take a deep breath in and count slowly to 5 as you breathe in and as you breathe in let your stomach rise for one, two, three and four, five and release and exhale as your stomach goes back down. Count your exhale one, two, three, four, five, six and seven release as you release your breath. Take another deep breath in as you rise your stomach and now hold your breath for, one, two, three, four, five counts, and release in your exhale as your body and stomach releases back down as you breathe to one, two, three, four, five, six and seven counts.

Feel the sensation of your body becoming lighter and lighter the more relaxed it has now become, you are feeling lighter and relaxed. Your body is feeling pure genuine love through the beautiful healing colors that are now penetrating your body. It is releasing natural healing molecules into your body, naturally, feel your body warming to the healing that is now taking place. You are healing, you are relaxed.

All your thoughts and attention is in a relaxed state of healing, you are allowing the healing energy and vibrational frequencies to release its healing molecules into your body. You are feeling so relaxed and blissful. Feel the beauteous healing colors of the sunset come through your feet, feel the sensation of its energy moving up through the bottom and front of your feet. Feel the healing colors move up through the back and front of your calves and knees as the healing colors are healing and energizing you with vibrant health, allowing your body to be in a state of healing and ease. See and feel the colors moving up through to your hips and buttocks area, feel the relaxation as the energy moves through your body. Focus and see the redish color moving through your body and up to your first energy centre the first chakra of your pelvic area of your body. See and feel the redish color balance and permeate the color red in your pelvic area, breathe in the red color to your pelvic area. You can do this to the in breath again of 5 counts and hold for five counts then release for seven counts. You can do this dame count for every energy chakra area.

Now see and feel just below your navel, your lower stomach area and see and feel the color bright orange color swirling through below your navel area. Feel the orange color as it relaxes more into your navel area and lower stomach. Breathe in the color orange in your navel area and lower stomach and back area and breathe out the orange color, feeling and knowing it's balancing the energy in your lower stomach. Feel the ease of digestion as the healing color of orange warms that area of your lower stomach, feel how well your digestion is working.

Move your attention and see and feel the color bright yellow color as it penetrates and moves through and above your navel and stomach area. See and feel as the bright sun shines it's healing and balancing on your 3rd energy centre, the 3rd chakra, see the yellow swirling color fill your stomach area just above your navel. See and feel the bright yellow color and breathe in yellow to that area while relaxing into it and exhale the yellow and allow your stomach to release and it goes down. Your lower stomach is relaxed in its bright yellow energy.

Move your attention and energy up to your heart area, the 4th energy chakra and see and feel the color emerald green vibrantly pulsating and penetrating your heart and lung area. Breathe in the emerald color green through your heart area and exhale the emerald color green and you release your breath. You body is so relaxed and allowing and accepting all healing, it is in its natural ease. Breathe in again the healing emerald green color to and through your heart area and exhale and release the color emerald green, knowing that your heart is of genuine pure love. You see love in everyone and everything, love is your divine birth rite, you are created from love, you are love. See and feel the emerald green color continue to relax your heart area.

Allow and feel while your attention moves up your body from your lungs and heart area and relax your spine and shoulders. Feel the ease and relaxation of your spine and shoulders and take a deep breath in while you extend and allow your stomach to rise and then release your breath as you exhale and allow your stomach to release and come down. Move your attention and love energy up through and to your throat area. See and feel the color of the sky blue as the puffy white clouds surround the sky you see the light sky blue radiating into your throat area, front and back and all around your throat area. See and feel and breathe in the sky light color blue and feel the blue color and energy relax and align to penetrate all healing and balancing energy to your throat area. Take a deep breath in while seeing the sky blue color swirling around your throat area and release with your exhale knowing your throat and vocals are always allowing your natural true expression of ease.

Move your attention and feel your chin on your face relaxed and your cheeks and neck relaxed and you take in another deep breath, inhale for five counts, one, two, three, four, five and release, exhale your breath for seven counts and allow your body to ease back on your exhale. Relax while moving your attention on your eyes, pure vision, you can see so clearly close and far. If any other thoughts try to intrude, tell them to go away and focus your attention on the healing of your body and now your eyes. Your eyes shine of love because that is what you are made out of, pure genuine divine love of our creator. Relax your eyes and take a deep breath in and exhale and you continue to be at ease of your whole body.

Move your attention up to the bridge of your nose in between your eye brows and see and feel the color indigo, the dark blue color of the night sky as it illuminates the stars to shine so bright just before it gets pitch dark. See and feel the dark blue color penetrate through the bridge of your nose between your eyebrow area. Take a deep inhale of the dark color blue as it penetrates the bridge area of the top of your nose. Allow the ease of your divine nature to release and ease the area. Take another deep breath in and hold for one, two, three and four, five now release your exhale in seven counts and relax even deeper.

Move your attention upwards to the top of your head and see and feel the violet purply color as the sunset is coming to its nightly peak. See and feel the purply color come through to the top of your head as it relaxes with ease your head allowing all genius to take root, seeded of your natural infinite intuition of wisdom. See and feel the purply violet color penetrate while it swirls through your head and top of you head front and back. Take a deep breath in as you see and feel the purply violet color ease your head and energizing your head with its divine nature and exhale and release your breath as you continue to be at ease and relax.

Move and keep your attention on the color gold as it surrounds and engulfs you with universal wisdom and see the bright white light protecting the whole of you. Just as icing is put on a cake you are allowing the bright light to energize and protect your body in its white pure light from your head, down your face and throat, shoulders and spine and neck through to your heart and lungs and stomach, buttocks to your pelvic area and legs, knees, calves front and back and feet. You are an extension of the infinite creator, you are love and you now know it.

You know the difference of your body being in ease and out of ease, whenever you think of your body and nature you think and feel health, ease, your body is always in a state of desiring ease and health. It becomes easier and easier for you to think and feel healthy, you know its natural for your body. It's easier for your body to be in a healed ease state when you keep your thoughts and feelings in the ease natural state. Take a deep breath in of five counts and then hold for five counts and then exhale for seven counts. Take another deep breath in as your stomach rises and hold and exhale, release your breath while your body and stomach releases against the floor. You now feel energized, filled with love and ease and health, you are healthy.

As you take another breath in feel yourself becoming aware and submerged in the present moment of now and your surroundings. Feel your eyes now opening and see how wonderful and miraculous everything really is, how you appreciate everything you see and encounter. See the sky and the sun has set and you feel renewed and refresh. Take one more deep breath in and then release with that renewed energized feeling. And know you are Love.

End of visualized imagining.

If you were to do this twice or at least once a day, I guarantee it would make quite the difference in how your body feels. It would also make a difference in how you will perceive everything in your life with more ease and love which we know ease and love is what creates and sustains a healthy body.

You can modify by changing a sunset to lying on a beach with the waves of the water or if you enjoy storms or snow, use whatever creates the most pleasure and joy for you when you set the scene for your imaginings. The more you do this the more you will be able to bring yourself in a meditative state or an imaginative state. Both are the same states, its all about focusing on one thing and keeping the focus of your attention on whatever you are desiring. Even when other nagging thoughts try to disturb you, you just accept it and let it go and focus back onto what you desire to focus your attention upon.

Throughout the day you can do mini imaginings, by just stopping and focusing your attention for a few minutes on the part of your body you want to heal. A few minutes a day really do add up and before you know it you will see improvement. The more you do it the easier it becomes, like a snap you will be in a healing state of focus. If old thoughts of doubt appear, by letting them go in love and inserting the thoughts and feelings as if you are already healed will become less and less resistant with doubt. When you can go along a whole day and whenever you think of your diseased or painful body spots without a doubt and just see and feel already healed, then you know you have changed. Your body is changing and soon what will follow is complete healing. I also suggest to not stop the imaginings once healed, use it for other things you want to heal or you desire to manifest. Let it become a daily habit and you will see your body and life change in amazing ways.

Chapter Seventeen

Your Heart and Bliss is the Key to DNA Changes in Self Healing

If you absolutely knew that staying in the feelings of bliss could cure and heal all diseases would you work on staying blissful through everything?

Knowledge about your heart, bliss and healing is the most important information you could ever know because of what occurs in your body when you stay blissful.

There is biological evidence now that supports when we stay blissful our body cells, organs and especially our heart performs from responding in bliss by creating a spin in our DNA that creates healing. You can check out any of Dan Winter's information on Bliss. This is the literal reason that staying blissful no matter what you are going through is what is going to change the information that becomes decoded within your DNA with information that creates the healing. There is an implosion that squirts out cascades of proteins of chemicals that creates the body to heal itself when you stay in the feelings of bliss. I wrote a whole book on bliss, "The Hidden Key Orgasm Reveals" its all about bliss and its benefits. Orgasm is actually our teacher when we understand the feelings that I believe orgasm was inherited in us originally and for its great use.

Bliss is our natural inherited gene in our DNA that becomes activated through the gathering of emotions into a cascade into feelings through our heart. It has always been there, however it's not taught of the importance bliss is or how to actually sustain bliss either.

So you who are reading this and resonating with this information is really on the leading edge, you will find soon in the future it will become evident. For now you must trust your intuition to believe it is true and experiment with healing and bliss so that you can know for yourself so that you no longer have any doubts.

In the teaching of visualizing or imaging yourself as already healed you will experience that when you are imagining for a long enough time that you bring yourself to feeling blissful. This is the biological reason that imagining works. It creates memories for you to retrieve while simultaneously your whole body and through your heart is responding by affecting your DNA and all your body cells.

Stop thinking your heart is just a pump that is pumping blood throughout your body and start thinking about your heart as a master genius part of your body. People who suffer with heart conditions are experiencing the end result of their heart communicating information. Anyone with heart problems has been allowing themselves to be slipping away from their joys and what they love in their life. They are hurting their heart by not feeling and following their joy of bliss.

We have all heard about one mate dying and then shortly after the other left behind becomes so heart broken and literally biologically affects the heart. Or a relationship ending, it's all the same thing separation from what the individual has put or invested so much joy and love into. Even if it was a negative or abusive relationship, the heart doesn't know the difference because in one's heart the person feels the connection and is still addicted to the other person. Altered love takes on many different forms and most individuals still does not know pure unaltered, unconditional love of bliss or that their love or loving is not pure. Most are still dealing with addictive love, this is another subject but it's important to know that lack of JOY. BLISS of love does affect the heart.

Our hearts can be filled with feelings of joyful bliss of pure love or with feelings of the opposite and you will always know the difference by being aware how you are feeling. Whether you feel blissful with unconditional connected love or are experiencing negative feelings that feel's the complete opposite which is separated from love.

Heredity and Genetics

We must keep in mind that heredity of genetics of diseases can be changed as Bruce Lipton's work has shown that heredity is more of a subconscious role modeling than anything else we have been taught to believe. If we believe the old teachings that if there is heart disease, or any disease in our family then we have created a belief that creates it to most likely carry it on and be affected by genetics.

Well the new information shows us this is all false information we invested unconsciously to believe. Instead when we respond differently to what is going on, that responding differently literally changes our genetic coding of information in our DNA. This then changes what we believed to be the cause of genetic diseases and will not create the disease that was thought in the past to be inevitable.

What empowering knowledge of information this is that we can change our DNA literally just by choosing thoughts that build on this powerful knowledge. This gives you the potential to perpetually affect your DNA and changes the genetics, the decoding of information. Just by choosing already healed thoughts that fuel feelings of optimism, love, trust and bliss that generate the chemicals in our body to transform so magically as a result.

If you still do not believe this then it's essential that you watch intensively on youtube of Bruce Lipton and Dan Winter. Extending the information into your own life to see the proof for yourself will totally transform all your old beliefs that has been dictating the wrong information your whole life.

Is it not worth the new work? You will do it if you really want to change and heal your body. If you do not then you will carry on in pain and allow the disease to take your over and could also prematurely end your life. The decision will always be up to you only.

It will take doing so many things differently in your life. Instead of spending hours doing something that is not in alignment with your new healing ways of thinking, you change it. By reading or listening to more information of present day wisdom of information that is available now through our amazing technology.

Or sit quietly and go within and receive your pure information without your old programs tainted with doubt. Or just become a love bliss transformer, meaning deliberately transforming everything to love and bliss because you just know in your heart, soul and spirit that its worth it and beneficial in every way.

Maybe that will be the inspiration that ignites the passion for the changes to become for you. Whatever it takes I guarantee you it's worth it, you will know for yourself and not have to be confused about anything any longer.

You will look in the mirror and naturally instantly love who you are because you came to know who you are, a loving infinite being experiencing physical reality. You may even become to know that love and bliss is your purposeful journey this lifetime and you will no longer alter from your love and bliss for anything or anyone.

You will know that this is the most loving way to be always and this way is not only healing yourself but the planet and everyone on it too. You will realize how we really are all connected and that love, bliss and unity is always the way.

Website

If you have any questions about what you have read in this book, you can ask or contact me through my website. Or if you have any healing experiences you would like to share with us, please do at the website on the self healing page. You may find other abilities and information that you might be interested in too.

http://www.infinite-manifesting.org/

Disclaimer

Even though I know most of you are already quite responsible for your own self to listen and take whatever resonates with you in all that you have read. I still must add a disclaimer that states the obvious; that I do not and will not be responsible for anything you have read or try from my information I am sharing with you. It works I know that! But if you go off your medication please only do what you know you are ready to do. I know this seems like common enough sense but it's still important that you realize that self healing takes going through the stages you need to go through when you are ready.

So in other words I am sharing my experiences honestly of what I have experienced and learned. It is totally your responsibility what you then do with it and I am not held responsible. This is the way it should be of course because whenever an individual evolves to become self responsible then these types of disclaimers really become obsolete. But then that would mean that we already live in a harmonious, connected world. Though we are on our way, we're not there yet and this is the reason I must write and add a disclaimer.

Suggested and Further Learning Information

Louise Hay Heal Your Life

Deepak Chopra Ageless Body, Timeless Mind

Martin Brofman http://www.healer.ch/

Dan Winter http://www.danwinter.com/

Bruce Lipton Biology of Belief

Wayne Dyer Excuses Begone

Gregg Braden http://www.greggbraden.com/

What the Bleep, Movie and website
http://www.whatthebleep.com/

Seth-Jane Roberts
The Nature of Personal Reality (Book)

The Living Matrix Movie
http://www.thelivingmatrixmovie.com/

What If? The Movie
http://www.whatifthemovie.tv/

Books by
AnnaMarie Antoski

Infinite Manifesting
Journey Within to Your Infinite Self

The Hidden Key Orgasm Reveals
Living a Blissful Life

Evolving Reality of Bewitched
Living a Magical Life

Stumbling through Infinity
Heart Reflection Poetry

Knowledge Transforms to Wisdom
Expanding Consciousness Poetry

Forever in Bloom
Combined Poetry Collection

Nature Abound

ABOUT THE AUTHOR

AnnaMarie Antoski has been her own self healer for over 20 years and has learned and taught others how to transform experiences into bliss and experience the benefits of self healing. She has consistently studied the nature of reality and has implemented all she has learned into her daily life and is on a continuous evolving journey of sovereignty.